Table of Contents

Impact of Addison's Disease on the Skin: Symptoms and Treatment

1. Introduction to Addison's Disease

The disease mostly affects people in their early 30s and 40s. Women are more commonly affected, and in 2008, the disease affected about 4 in 100,000 people. The condition usually presents in those over 30 to 50 years but can present at any age. People with Addison's disease or family members who have the condition or other autoimmune diseases are more likely to develop Addison's disease. An autoimmune disease causes the body to attack its own tissues, causing inflammation and harm. It is not clear what makes the immune system attack the adrenal glands, and also lead to other autoimmune disorders such as ovarian tumors, thyroid disease, type 1 diabetes, and underactive parathyroid glands. Infections, such as tuberculosis, histoplasmosis, or CMV, can damage the adrenal glands. It is possible to have this type of the disorder after a cancerous growth in the adrenal glands is surgically removed. Hemorrhage or blood clots into the adrenal glands also cause it, as do other physical stresses, such as severe burns, infections or other illnesses. Adrenal insufficiency can happen because of opiates taken for long periods, such as morphine, or synthetic opioids medications such as oxycodone. In sufferers of acquired immunodeficiency syndrome (AIDS) risk of adrenal insufficiency increases because of infections such as cytomegalovirus, AIDS-related fungal infections, or mycobacterial infections such as tuberculosis in the adrenal glands. The disease is infrequent in the United States and is included in the orphan disorders.

Addison's disease occurs when the adrenal cortex is damaged and the adrenal glands do not produce sufficient cortisol (or corticosteroid) and, to varying degrees, aldosterone. The primary form of the disease is generally caused by the body attacking itself (autoimmune), and the secondary form is when the pituitary gland does not produce an adequate supply of the hormone that stimulates the production of cortisol. A common presentation is dark pigmentation and vitiligo, although in the earlier stages this can be non-specific.

1.1. Definition and Overview

The condition is managed through lifetime steroid replacement treatment, which mimics the contours of cortisol produced by healthy adrenal glands. Without treatment, a person may become seriously unwell and can potentially die. Regardless of the presence of skin abnormalities in approximately 90% of patients, not all of them are employed as a diagnostic tool. Hence, there is growing interest in the study of numerous skin manifestations in patients with Addison's disease: from changes in pigmentation—considered to be one of the clinical manifestations of primary adrenal insufficiency, as stated by the fifth President of the US, Abraham Lincoln "[b]oth labia and beard are flaxen, and skin very white"—to disorders of sebocytes, melanocytes or increased hair growth due to androgen deficiency. In fact, there seems to be a major unsolved problem organizing the complexity of skin alterations in primary adrenal insufficiency and its related studies.

Addison's disease is a rare endocrine condition caused by the malfunction of the human adrenal glands. More specifically, primary Addison's disease (the focus of this review) is a state of adrenal insufficiency resulting from damage to the adrenal glands. In the countries where population studies are available, there have been 39 and 60 cases identified in 2011 in the UK and the United States, respectively, with around 1 in 10,000 people or more affected by this rare endocrine condition. Although considered rare, with growing difficulties of definitive diagnosis, we may begin to understand that this disorder may not be as rare as once thought.

1.2. Causes and Risk Factors

Addison's disease is the result of infections, thrombosis, hemochromatosis, other glandular destruction, malignancies, and other causes. And the CECS diagnosis can be attempted if signs and symptoms are detected. Although Addison's disease is a systemic disease, patients with skin involvement should be under the care of dermatologists. However, no research had been performed on the occurrence as well as the effect on the skin until the present research. This review article was aimed at identifying symptoms as well as the types of skin modifications in the event of Addison's disease. In addition, the report would be a good help for dermatologists attempting to manage patients with suspected Addison's disorders, and dermatologists and psychologists could treat these patients in outpatient settings.

Addison's disease is a rare idiopathic primary adrenal insufficiency associated with selective autoimmune destruction of the adrenal cortex. Symptoms of skin changes appear as hyperpigmentation of the skin with some distribution and are usually dominant on the knees, hand lines, or elbows. Skin hyperpigmentation has different influences such as urinary accession and Kaposi-Juliusberg dermatitis. The presenting symptom of Addison's disease in chronic form is hyperpigmentation of the face and hands, with or without fatigue. The chronic form is characterized by gradually worsened symptoms accompanied by a variety of clinical and laboratory abnormalities. The chronic form has been described primarily in women aged 20-40 years, but it can occur at any age. Granulomatosis usually occurs as chronic inflammation of an adrenal insufficiency as primary or secondary endocrine disorders, and most are caused by tuberculosis and non-infectious granuloma or polyglandular autosomal syndromes (APS) except tuberculous adrenalitis. On imaging, the adrenal glands are usually normal or small. Infection by Mycobacterium tuberculosis is diagnosed by culture, PCR, and steroid testing, by comparing lymphocytes of Pleural and ascitic fluidex.

By: 1) Division of Dermatology, University Hospital "Gaetano Martino", 98122 Messina, Italy 2) Dermatology Unit, Department of Clinical Medicine, University of Insubria, ASST dei Sette Laghi, 21100 Varese, Italy

2. Skin Manifestations of Addison's Disease

The most frequent cutaneous feature is diffuse or spotted hyperpigmentation. Less frequent cutaneous features of Addison's disease include diffuse hypopigmentation, vitiligo, psoriasiform eruptions, sarcoidlike plaques, scrotal tongue, alopecias, pruritus, vitiligo, atrophic scars, Henoch-Schönlein-like purpura, livedo reticularis, livedo racemosa, cutis marmorata, anetoderma, erythroderma, capillary angiomas, pruritus, urticaria, flushing, hypo- or hyperthermia, erythema, venous leg ulceration, dermatitis, keloids, collagenoma, cutis laxa, striae atrophicae, atopic dermatitis, ichthyosis, prurigo, papules and ulcers, hyperkeratoses, urticaria pigmentosa, mastocytomas, Darier's sign. Itching, scaling, and dryness of the skin are highly common and found in about 70% of the reported cases. Various hair changes such as excessive hair shedding, loss of body hair, thinning, or graying of scalp hair have been reported. On the other hand, there are also less frequent side effects of adrenal insufficiency, like hypertrichosis and androgenic alopecia in men. Patients with clinical signs of chronic adrenocortical insufficiency may present to various specialists; hence cutaneous features of the disease are important clues for correct diagnosis and treatment.

The skin, being the largest organ in the body, is often a mirror of the underlying internal diseases. Addison's disease was the first disease to be associated with the skin.

Addison's disease is characterized by the insufficient production of aldosterone and cortisol by the adrenal glands. Chronic adrenocortical insufficiency due to destruction or dysfunction of the adrenal cortex is known as "Addison's disease," first described by Thomas Addison in 1855. It has a wide diversity of cutaneous features which have been recognized over the last century and are associated with increased morbidity.

2.1. Hyperpigmentation

Given that redheads do not burn out easily, another reason is their minor level of choroidal pigmented melanocytes, whereas most brown spots do not appear to produce them that quickly and simply. Except in a congenital disorder, the choroid melanins are stable in position. Proopiomelanocortin is dramatically increased in the ACTH dependent classic adrenal insufficiency so that it stimulates pigmentation over the complete pituitary and central nervous system.

Hyperpigmentation is a hallmark clinical feature of Addison's disease, though it can also develop with some regularity in patients with the chronic form of the condition. It is not just a tan. Despite an increase in production of skin pigment, the response to appropriate sunshine, or the turnstile for pigment-manufacturing sun rays, is not bypassed. Tanning and pigmentation normally develop after the immediate response is artificially altered. This is partly because regular sunlight travels through a granular layer of the skin, stimulating a surge of the pigment manufactory, melanocytes. The resulting melanocytes must go somewhere once they are made, and the melanocytes serve the increased population. This is key to the autonomic cycle of melanin synthesis and helps to direct our focus on pigmentation diagnosis, a clear example of skin involvement.

2.2. Hypopigmentation

All therapies that are aimed at dealing with the hypopigmentation focus mainly on the zona glomerulosa deficiency. Dosages of up to 1.2 mg/day of fludrocortisone will, if anything, reduce the risk of hypotension and increase the plasma sodium concentration. This may nourish, but not stimulate, the melanocytes. In general, administration of up to 0.3 mg/day of fludrocortisone or only the administration of hydrocortisone up to 20 mg/day does not completely prevent Addisonian orthostatic hypotension. Only a minor percutaneous absorption of fludrocortisone is needed for Miner's disease treatment. Further important reasons for the return of pigmentation are the normalization of adrenocorticotropin hormone and concentration, and also that the administration of fludrocortisone and hydrocortisone coincides with sunlight.

A considerable hypopigmentation of the skin is often mentioned in patients with Addison's disease. This finding might be because of tolerance to sun exposure and the accompanying reduced functioning of the melanocytes. In the photographs showing Jonathan Kennedy with his hypopigmented skin, the elbows, knees, and face are less pigmented than the normal skin, with irregular areas of hyper- and depigmentation on both elbows. The irregular distribution of depigmented and normally pigmented skin is consistent with a focal vitiligo-like depigmentation. Reintgen also notes a significant response vis-à-vis the restoration of pigment with fludrocortisone treatment in his patients. Habek and Bastaić also interpreted the hypopigmentation as irreversible sun damage superimposed on the loss of normal pigmentation. Of special interest is the absence of lentigines both on the skin of Jonathan Kennedy and on Aurélien, who has had long-standing Addison's disease from an unknown etiology. The medical literature shows that Addison's disease in general predisposes to increased formation and pigmentation of lentigines.

2.3. Dryness and Scaling

Dryness of the skin manifests itself by brittleness as well as by desquamation. The skin might also become fissured, particularly in the flexural areas of the body such as the epiganthic fold, groin region, and axillas because of the repeated stretching movements. The compositions of the perspiration, sebum, and hydrolipidic mantle are further modified, giving an altered pleasant odour to the already dark tanned skin. The severity of the skin manifestations might therefore reflect the amount of general hyperpigmentation to result in black palmar hand dermatitis. All these skin manifestations not only give a poor cosmetic image but also contribute to the risks of local infectious complications as well as to an overall disfiguring dermatitis.

The skin is the most exposed organ of the human body and is also the first visible manifestation to the world. Skin signs and symptoms are the second most common complaint about the skin due to altered mineralocorticoid homeostasis in Addison's disease. Dry skin and increased transcutaneous water loss are most commonly seen as an early feature due to hypocortisolism. Chronic salt craving or reduced oral salt intake leads to hyperkalemia, which causes the typical salt-craving dermatitis known as "toffee" coloured hyperkeratosis. In contrast, the chronic loss of mineralocorticoid effect leads to increased production of adrenocorticotrophic hormone, which in turn causes an increase in the expression of melanocyte stimulating hormone (a-MSH). The expression of MSH has been identified not only in the infundibula keratinocytes but also in the eccrine and apocrine ducts, which might explain the increased hair pigmentation in generalized forms of the disease.

2.4. Hair Changes

Addison's disease is associated with progressively decreasing density of body hair. The hair is also normal in calorific production depending on the maintenance intake of thyroid hormone. The pigmentation in vitiligo patches and all of the hair follicles will decrease as the patches become larger. This reduction, related to the intrafollicular estrogen- and/or cortisol-related proteolytic enzyme neutral metalloproteinase, appears to also interfere with the normal hair cycle. Consequently, in addition to atrophy and lower activation of vitiliginous hair follicles, the growth phase of non-vitiliginous hair follicles becomes longer. Overall, the latter phenomenon results in increased growth of unaffected hair and decreased shedding. Signs of skin surface MI. Additionally, occasional yellowish discoloration of the skin caused by xanthomas, fatty deposits in the connective tissue, may occur. As long as the connective tissue is involved, it may also infiltrate abnormal mitochondria in order to detect the Hartnup disease gene for liver enzymes. Skin biopsies are used in very few patients to verify the diagnosis and assess the course of the disease.

The hair of many patients with Addison's disease is dry, brittle, coarser, and may tangle easily. Because of the dryness, the ability of hair to mount an electrical charge is diminished, and the hair may become lank and may not cling to the scalp. The changes are more pronounced in lightly pigmented individuals. Patients usually do not suffer from baldness. The hair may grow more slowly than normal. However, in general, the patient's hair may recover relatively quickly with appropriate steroids. Sex hormones are also related to these abnormalities.

3. Diagnosis and Assessment of Skin Symptoms

All mites, ticks, head lice (pediculosis), and skin fleas should be killed.

Management of infestations

Based on the history and clinical presentation, the findings of blood cultures confirm spirochete infections from: Borrelia for Borreliosis Streptobacillus monilsformisisoides (rat bite fever, Haverhill fever) and Streptobacillus notomytis, both rare pathological relapsing fever Borrelia, are unique in agricultural practices that can result in human infection from. The post-treatment chemical reaction of Warthin-Starri stain serves no diagnostic function. Positive serology for other agents is a good indication that spirochetes other than Borrelia have induced the systemic development of these symptoms. Acute hemolytic anemia may be diagnostic. False positive VDRL and weak 2ME tests are frequently obtained. For microbiological bugs, microscopic agglutination testing is very specific. The VDRL is generally reactive, but a nontreponemal test doesn't identify Borrelia disease. Crithidia positive immunofluorescence assays can provide proof of Borrelia disease faster than other tests. Serologies rely on seroconversion over weeks or longer. Titration is used for serodiagnosis. Due to sensitivity issues, seronegative reactions are unusual. Borrelia may be the differential diagnosis in the context of continuing symptoms. The urine OspA test, which is omitted here, could be a valuable early diagnostic biomarker.

Diagnosis

The historical evaluation of athletes, arthropod exposure, and existing scalp and body makeup are necessary for recognition. Because systemic reactions are critical, the diagnosis of crustacean allergy and tick-borne relapsing fever should be evaluated. The Tibetan region, Africa-crimes, and Latin America are all endemic areas for human relapsing fever. The skin and fascia are deeply involved. The possibility exists for fly-bites to transmit relapsing fever through infected agriculture. Typically, skin manifestations serve as hallmarks for diagnosis and treatment to guarantee prompt management. In patients with Addison's disease, skin manifestations are seen long after illness begins, as are varicella-like papulovesicular skin lesions progressing to full-thickness necrosis and eschar at puncture sites, face, and extremities. Abscesses can form deep in the soft tissues. Subclinical cases of cutaneous leishmaniasis can cause a TT-positive skin test. Congenital immune disorders associated with increased susceptibility to disease are evidence of late death following live viral vaccinations.

Clinical Evaluation

4. Treatment Options for Skin Manifestations

Topical corticosteroids are often the frontline treatment for rashes and other skin conditions. They are not absorbed into the rest of the body, in general, and can be applied as often as needed. They are for sale in pharmacies without a prescription and come in a variety of concentrations and preparations. Oral corticosteroids are also very useful for many people with chronic rashes and skin conditions. They are available with a prescription and allow us to attack and control the underlying disease process directly. This has advantages in some cases but also serious disadvantages. The most dangerous is that they can either trigger the onset of symptoms that never before developed or cause long-dormant symptoms to come back with a vengeance. Fortunately, they are typically not a mainstay of management and can be avoided in most cases. They are for sale in pharmacies without a prescription, although there are few with that indication. Be sure to talk to a doctor beforehand. Moisturizers are critical for skin problems at all times when many are used with other treatments and can help with difficulty healing. They are available for sale everywhere. Topical corticosteroids often work best when they are applied directly after applying a moisturizer. Retinols, alpha hydroxy acids, and other cosmetic remedies can do more harm than good and are typically not recommended. Massage often helps. Heat therapy often helps. Emollients are often useful and can be found in products with other active ingredients.

There are many active treatments available that can be used to directly address the effects of Addison's disease at a dermatological level, mainly for the skin conditions that are rarely noticed by those with it. These treatments are not curative; none are curative and none of the damage can be reversed. These treatments help to keep some of the effects at bay, delaying the point at which they may develop further or progress. For that reason, they are necessarily designed to be used for the remainder of life.

4.1. Topical Corticosteroids

4.1.1. Mechanism of Action Topical corticosteroids have been used in many diseases and for the treatment of symptoms seen in so many other illnesses. Cutaneous manifestations of Addison's disease can be treated with very high potency topical corticosteroid. In contrast, oral corticosteroids can often have systemic side effects which should be avoided, particularly in patients with mild symptoms. Strong topical steroids have the potential to cause systemic side effects, but these are much less likely than with oral steroids. Potent topical steroids have a very potent local anti-inflammatory effect. Topical formulations of corticosteroids can act through inhibiting the production of proinflammatory cytokines such as interleukin (IL)-1. Efficacy of treatment has been seen within days and with definitive results within a matter of weeks.

It is generally considered that topical corticosteroids are of little use in the treatment of systemic Addison's disease. However, when skin manifestations are not systemic, but present as an isolated finding, then the use of topical therapies may be more acceptable. Topical corticosteroids remain the mainstay of treatment as they should, in part, act as a targeted steroid administration. Their rationale is not to replace or replicate the loss of glucocorticoid hormones, but rather targeted toward the potential immunosuppressive function which may alleviate specific dermatological symptoms.

4.2. Oral Corticosteroids

Despite the widespread belief that glucocorticoid replacement leads to improvement of skin symptoms, there is a lack of contemporary data defining the corticosteroids that are most effective and ideal replacement strategies in those with active eczema. Clarification is warranted to optimize outcomes for patients with significant skin morbidity in this field. Addison's disease (AD) is a rare condition characterized by primary hypofunction of the adrenal glands with typical symptoms of hyponatremia, hyperkalemia, and pressure collapse. Skincare in primary adrenal deficiency includes the regular, consistent use of emollients and treatment of eczema with mild to moderate-strength corticosteroids.

Mild to moderate glucocorticoid insufficiency is commonly treated with hydrocortisone replacement therapy, although available clinical data do not describe in great detail the skin manifestations of Addison's disease and their response to glucocorticoid therapy. Results from our systematic review suggest that data on the effects of replacement therapy with oral corticosteroids in patients with skin symptoms are limited due to the rarity of the condition, heterogeneity of the participants, low methodological quality, inconsistencies in outcomes presentation, and the effect of different measures of the skin response on the methodological data. It further describes the results and additional adverse events. In conclusion, the use of oral corticosteroids in patients with skin manifestations of primary hypoadrenalism is more of a single case management approach, necessitating close patient monitoring for infection, hyperglycemia, deleterious effects on the skin, as well as possible further skin deterioration (e.g., thinning and bruising).

4.3. Moisturizers and Emollients

Topical treatments can rectify the barrier structural alterations seen in cortisol deficiency. Chronic in vitro exposure to high doses of glucocorticoid has also been shown to significantly reduce the quantity and distribution of aquaporin-3 in human keratinocytes, which reduces water release to the cutaneous surface, replenishing contents of epidermal keratinocytes. They have also shown increased production of proteases that can further redistribute and cause secretion of signaling cytokines and chemokines involved in early cell-cell and cell-extracellular matrix interactions required for healing. Therefore, treatment with glucocorticoid can partially reverse these changes and may alleviate these pathogenic processes. Also, using a dermal infuser (ultrasound-assisted drug delivery), Sculptra can be given with much less skin irritation, providing face volume, and for very bad cases that could cause necrosis of the skin. It is recommended to avoid soap, especially in very dry skin. Soap contains fatty lye, and long-term use can dry the skin. A 'soap substitute' like Aveeno, Hydromol, or Oilatum seems to be effective, which can wash and moisturize the skin. Although strong soaps or shower gels are suitable when the skin is very oily, they are not recommended as they may disturb the barrier. Regular use of very greasy shower gels on the body or astronomical amounts of skincare on the face can cause folliculitis, which is difficult to manage.

Dryness is actually one of the most commonly reported symptoms that is bettered by treatment in some case reports. Patients tend to report dry (38%) or less commonly oily skin (9%), although in clinical studies, the reported incidence of dry skin is less (4%). Overt dryness has been reported as a cause of non-compliance with corticosteroid replacement, and 31% of patients attending a specialist clinic found that their skin condition influenced which doses of steroid they took as required. Symptoms associated with dry skin include scaling, pain, and pruritus, as well as an actual dry and wrinkled appearance. The main role of adjunctive care in dryness-related skin changes is to reduce dry cracking and scaling and to reduce any associated pruritus and pain. When choosing a moisturizer, it is logical to consider the main cause of dryness in Addison's, namely cortisol deficiency. Cortisol has an anti-inflammatory effect on the skin, particularly seen in the loss of elasticity and other changes that result from dermal inflammation and thinning, apart from normalizing epithelial barrier factors.

5. Conclusion and Future Directions

Much study of the cell cycle is needed to develop an understanding of the mechanisms behind skin fibrosis in Addison's disease. Patients who manifest with hypopigmentation or dyspigmentation of the skin could benefit from future research on melanoblast and melanocyte stem cell activation. Scarring or dermal atrophy are symptoms manifesting from depletion of epidermal stem cells, and therefore future research could investigate melanocyte stem cell and epidermal stem cell deletion in response to stress in the hyperstimulation of cortisol. The effect of changes in temperature of extremities via glucocorticoids is an interesting area of research as there appear to be emotional triggers to elephant hands. There is still much to learn regarding cellular dysfunction in Addison's disease.

In conclusion, this review highlights our current understanding of the role of cortisol in the skin and changes to skin structure and morphology observed in patients with Addison's disease. It is therefore illustrated that skin conditions commonly manifest as presenting or additional symptoms of Addison's disease and can be the primary issue for patients rather than other systemic disturbances. In cases when skin cell migration is dependent on glucocorticoids, patients who are untreated, diagnosed with an illness, or suffering emotional stress, which increases their cortisol clearance, can portray any of the symptoms highlighted in this paper.

The Comprehensive Guide to Addison's Disease: Symptoms, Diagnosis, and Treatment

1. Introduction to Addison's Disease

The adrenal glands are found near the kidney in the upper back. The two adrenal glands look like flattened triangles and each one has two separate parts with different functions. The outer part, called the cortex, produces mineralocorticoids that help control blood pressure, glucocorticoids that control blood sugar levels, and some sex hormone precursors. The inner part, called the medulla, makes hormones that help us cope with stress. Addison's disease occurs when at least 90% of both adrenal glands have been destroyed. The adrenal cortex can be damaged centrally or peripherally, or both. Central damage occurs when the pituitary gland and the hypothalamus in the brain do not make sufficient cortisol-stimulating hormone or corticotrophin-releasing hormone. Peripheral damage occurs because of autoimmune damage, hemorrhage or other causes that may involve just one adrenal gland. In Western countries, Australia and New Zealand, most cases of Addison's disease are due to an underlying autoimmune process that leads to adrenal insufficiency.

Addison's disease is a condition that arises when the body's adrenal gland is not producing sufficient hormones. The adrenal glands are triangular-shaped organs located over the kidneys. The adrenal glands produce a number of hormones, which are essential for life and critical to a human's ability to cope with stress. When someone has Addison's disease, their adrenal glands are damaged, which means that they are unable to produce these stress hormones (corticosteroids). Without these critical hormones, Addison's disease can be life-threatening. Addison's disease is a rare disorder that affects around 0.8 in 10,000 people.

2. Anatomy and Function of the Adrenal Glands

All of these functions are vital to correctly understand in order to be aware of what happens in Addison's Disease, but the first two functions in particular – the role of the adrenal glands in mineral balance and in producing steroid hormones – are most important to explore in relation to this condition. Its use in managing operations of mineral metabolism and research to determine the pathogenesis, detection, and causes of chronic adrenal insufficiency are required to provide a better understanding of the process. The exponential rise in the knowledge of adrenal diseases and the appropriate approach to the diagnosis and care of adrenal patients is essential for this. The adrenal glands, along with this know-how, are now well-recognized for their role as an important endocrine organ in the balance and regulation of fat and energy consumption. They secrete numerous hormones directly into the crucial bloodstream that maintain homeostasis within the body, including cortisol, also known as cortisone, insulin, and adrenaline.

The adrenal glands are a pair of triangle-shaped structures that are positioned on top of each kidney. They weigh approximately 4-5 grams and are responsible for releasing several essential hormones such as cortisone, adrenaline, and aldosterone, among others. The cortices of the adrenal glands are responsible for the secretion of cortisone as well as aldosterone, while the adrenal medullae are responsible for the release of adrenaline, noradrenaline, and dopamine hormones. Through this mechanism, the adrenal glands are a critical part of the sympathetic and parasympathetic nervous systems, helping to regulate essential bodily functions such as mineral balance and stress response.

3. Causes and Risk Factors of Addison's Disease

Adrenal insufficiency secondary to processes that inhibit the adrenal glands' ability to release hormones is sometimes referred to as secondary adrenal insufficiency. According to the researchers, lacerations of adrenal veins are a frequent cause. Adrenal hemorrhage is a severe illness that can cause shock and, if not treated quickly, is often fatal. Another cause of primary adrenal insufficiency is an autoimmune response. Autoimmune polyglandular syndrome, which often includes other autoimmune disorders, or isolated adrenal disease may develop as a result of the immune response. Genetic mutations of one of the several proteins involved in the formation of hormones and the response to ACTH signaling could cause primary adrenal insufficiency. Familial glucocorticoid deficiency and triple A syndrome are two rare genetic disorders that fall under this category.

An autoimmune reaction triggers the majority of cases of primary adrenal insufficiency. In these cases, the body's immune system mistakenly attacks the outer layer of the adrenal gland, the adrenal cortex. The adrenal glands produce hormones that help the body stay healthy and respond to stress. The most commonly affected layer of the adrenal cortex is the adrenal cortex. Up to 80% of patients with autoimmune adrenalitis have autoantibodies to an enzyme involved in the synthesis of adrenal hormones, 21-hydroxylase. Primary adrenal insufficiency may also result from surgical removal of the adrenal glands or other conditions that destroy the adrenal glands or block the release of hormones. Tuberculosis and HIV/AIDS are examples of these.

4. Clinical Presentation and Symptoms of Addison's Disease

The skin often reflects a nutritional state and therefore, in a number of diseases, changes in the hair and epidermal appendages occur. In Addison's disease, the most notable symptom is brownish discoloration of the skin or biologically significant increase in pigmentation. In healthy human adults, skin is generally about 1.6 mm thick. Despite its apparent insignificance in the body compared with other body tissues, the skin forms the boundary between the inside and the outside of the body and plays a vital role in preserving bodily integrity. In total, skin abnormalities have been recorded in around 90% of patients with adrenal insufficiency. The researchers describe the skin as bloodless in prematurely aged and dead Addison patients.

In its early stages, Addison's disease symptoms are usually non-specific and individuals may not notice any obvious changes. The clinical oddities are exacerbated by the fact that the symptoms are often not uniform—different patients may display completely different complaints while still having the same disease. Laboratory parameters can also be used as a means of determining whether the patient has a deficiency. Addison's disease is a disorder involving a disrupted development of symptoms, usually from nonspecific complaints that appear a long time before the occurrence of acute adrenal insufficiency symptoms. Classification of the signs and symptoms seen in Addison's disease is generally used to facilitate reference and may include various categories of signs and symptoms.

4.1. Distinct Skin Effects

The second form of cutaneous involvement is usually associated with hyponatremia. It occurs due to increased secretion of antidiuretic hormone (ADH) which allows for an age-related increased number of melanocytic nevi, also known as moles on the skin. With decreased cortisol, the interference with vitamin D pathway may lead to alopecia. However, this is usually seen in long-term deficiency and is reversible with the administration of corticosteroid supplements. Given all these effects, it is no surprise that people with Addison's disease need to protect themselves well from the sun. Sunscreen is an excellent solution for many people, and with so many different options available, it should be easy to find the right one that fits your lifestyle. The weather, the amount of sun exposure you'll be getting, and your skin type are all important factors to consider when picking out the perfect sunscreen.

Addison's disease can exhibit dermatological manifestations in at least two forms. The first form of cutaneous involvement occurs due to increased levels of adrenocorticotropic hormone (ACTH) from the pituitary glands due to the absence of negative feedback, which leads to increased melanocyte-stimulating hormone released by the pituitary. The hormone stimulates melanocytes to produce a large amount of melanin, and it is directly responsible for the brown color. This brown discoloration is most visible in sun-exposed areas such as the face and hands. On the other hand, the non-exposed areas are not much affected. This phenomenon is termed primary melanism and appears to be reversible with the use of corticosteroid supplements, given at the right time and right dose. As the melanocytes are usually functioning during the reproductive stage, primary melanism is rarely seen in post-reproductive years.

5. Diagnosis and Differential Diagnosis

A patient with clinical suspicion of adrenal insufficiency should be assessed in two steps. The first test is the basal early morning cortisol concentrations. A cortisol level of > 150 nmol/L almost excludes adrenal insufficiency, while a cortisol level of > 500 nmol/L is consistent with an intact stimulated adrenal function. Patients who are taking medications interfering with cortisol measurements or have a risk of imminent adrenal crisis (shock, severe dehydration, or severe symptoms and signs suggestive of adrenal insufficiency such as hyperkalemia) should be assessed on clinical grounds alone and treatment commenced promptly.

Diagnosis. Addison's disease. With high suspicion of Addison's disease, morning cortisol levels < 100 nmol/L can be considered diagnostic, confirmed by elevated levels of adrenocorticotropic hormone (ACTH) if not already initiated. Correcting the cortisol cut-off level for the time of sampling / cortisol circadian rhythm, the type and immunoassay method should be considered for increased accuracy (Chapter 3 "Cortisol", and Chapter 8 "The hypothalamic – pituitary – adrenal axis"). Differential diagnosis in suspected identifying primary or secondary/tertiary adrenal failure is usually relatively easy, excluding iatrogenic adrenal insufficiency in those who are on steroids. The more challenging differential diagnostic step is to determine the cause of the adrenal insufficiency. The results from further dynamic testing, imaging and additional laboratory testing including autoantibodies, complemented by genetic testing, will guide this work-up.

6. Laboratory Tests and Imaging Studies

- For adrenal CR deposits, CT will have equivalent diagnostic value or greater than MRI. - Standard MRI has equivalent negative predictive value to CT in identifying hypopituitarism, but dynamic MRI adds greater positive predictive value. - Special considerations need to be taken as these studies are not easily reproducible and are not widely available. - Dynamic MRI (consists of a sequence of images taken at a particular site over a period of 4 to 6 minutes following IV contrast injection; this is the calculated time needed for the contrast to arrive at the portal circulation) allows for a distinction between delayed contrast enhancement of residual healthy pituitary tissue (if any) with early rapid drainage of the contrast from the small remaining gland in the absolute absence of the pituitary gland. - Clinical pituitary testing (CPTT) using variable and continuous metyrapone measures at 8 and 12 h is predictive of the result of other gold standard testing for the diagnosis of central adrenal insufficiency.

Imaging: Imaging studies are performed to seek alternative concurrent diagnoses suspected Diagnosis of secondary adrenal insufficiency and cortisol adequacy:

- Adrenal Autoantibody (AAA) testing has no role in the routine diagnostic work-up of Addison's disease.

Diagnostic Imaging

Cosyntropin stimulation test: Measurement of 250µg ACTH 1-24 synthetic analogue with an adequate cortisol response after 30 or 60 minutes.

Plasma ACTH concentrations: In primary adrenal insufficiency, plasma ACTH concentration is elevated. ACTH level should be interpreted with caution, as a low ACTH does not preclude the presence of primary adrenal insufficiency in the face of clinical adrenal insufficiency.

- ACTH/Basal Serum Cortisol ratio: The ACTH/Basal serum cortisol ratio of >100 confirms the presence of primary adrenal insufficiency and obviates any further dynamic tests. The ACTH/Basal serum cortisol ratio may be utilized to help identify subclinical hypocortisolism. For a ratio > 0.8, perform Cosyntropin stimulation test.

- Diagnosis of primary adrenal insufficiency: Measurement of basal serum cortisol concentration ≤ 100 nmol/L (3.5 µg/dL) confirms the diagnosis of adrenal insufficiency. If the basal serum cortisol is >150 nmol/L (5.5 µg/dL), adrenal insufficiency is unlikely. In the "grey zone" between 100-150 nmol/L, additional tests are needed.

Laboratory Tests

7. Treatment Options for Addison's Disease

Treatment options: 1. Drink plenty of fluids and eat a healthy diet. In case of dehydration or an illness, it is important to compensate for lost nutrients. 2. Wear a Medic Alert bracelet or necklace. It will inform health care providers about your condition in case of an emergency. If you have symptoms of Addison's disease, your doctor will take your medical history, order a series of laboratory tests, and guide your treatment plan based on the results. Your endocrinologist could conduct blood and urine tests to measure the level of hormones secreted and excreted by the adrenal glands. Tests may also determine if the adrenal glands are damaged. A blood test will help measure the levels of potassium, sodium, glucose, and adrenocorticotropic hormone (ACTH) in your blood. A test for potassium levels in the blood is essential. Cortisol and aldosterone can also be tested using blood samples. The patient will be asked to provide a 24-hour urine sample for testing. This includes collections of urine overnight and reviews the next day. It will check the cortisol secreted by the body. A future test will also be carried out at night and early in the morning to check the levels of cortisol in your system. Plasma renin helps to confirm the body's hormonal imbalances. A technician will be required to perform renin tests on blood samples taken during the day, in the early morning, and in the evening. It will also be taken overnight. A pregnancy test will also be carried out to exclude other ectopic hormonal conditions. The abuleit's determination should not be carried out if a pregnant woman has Addison's disease. Your doctor will develop a blood test schedule that works for you and determine the best course of treatment. The goal of treating Addison's disease is to replace the missing hormones. Once the treatment plan has been put into place, you may need to make occasional visits to your endocrinologist or a hospital to report your progress. You may need to have blood drawn so that your endocrinologist can check your potassium and sodium levels and adjust your medication if necessary. If you think you may need additional care and treatment, please report it to your endocrinologist or physician. It is best to receive treatment at a local health facility where the staff is familiar with you and your medical history. We will consult with the department on how to confirm the diagnosis.

There is no cure for Addison's disease, but there are several options for treating it. The focus of treatment for Addison's disease is to replace the hormones. Treatment involves addressing the cause of the deficiency. There is no way to prevent an Addison's crisis. The U.S. Food and Drug Administration has approved some hormonal replacement therapies. Prednisone should be the top choice because it improves aldosterone deficiency. If you lost weight or have low blood pressure, you might be prescribed hydrocortisone. Symptoms should be controlled with an adequate replacement dose. Additional medication is not needed. If your symptoms persist, consult your doctor. Certain hormone secretions from the adrenal glands or hormones released by the other parts of the adrenal glands are protected from the effects of cortisol. The hypothalamus secretes corticotropin-releasing hormone and the pituitary gland secretes adrenocorticotropic hormone. These are released as part of the body's stress response when cortisol levels are lower than normal. In case of emergencies, this helps to keep cortisol levels normal. Diabetics need to increase their dosage during an illness or an emergency surgery. If a person with Addison's disease becomes ill or has an operation, they need to seek medical attention. They may be prescribed intravenous (IV), a medication or a hospital stay.

7.1. Hormone Replacement Therapy

Commonly, neither dehydroepiandrosterone nor androgens are given as part of hormone replacement. There is no body of evidence that shows their absence at the levels found in health is somehow ill. Little is known about whether menstruants lose more corticosteroid during menstruation, the body using more cortisol in a cleverer way, or the body uses the same amount with production falling (or increasing) even more. Nevertheless, in more ill (worse quality of life) Addison's disease menstruants, we offer 5-10 mg hydrocortisone daily in the manner of cortisol secretion during rigors. Is it the corticosteroids, the mineralocorticoid, or the androgens in hormonal replacement that cures at least the worst tiredness of Addison's disease? Or is it the whole big "ball" that does the trick? If one makes a ball from cortisol, fludrocortisone, and testosterone, will this ball bring life quality matching that of the asymptomatic controls? The modern consensus on steroid replacement therapy has built up and is why and how we expect cortisol (or cortisone orally) and fludrocortisone acetate (if deficient, in amounts that reduce but do not abolish plasma renin activity), but not testosterone for adult females.

In hormone replacement therapy, patients receive the missing hormones in quantities that compensate for their adrenal insufficiency. Cortisol replacement, such as oral hydrocortisone or oral cortisone acetate, is necessary, pleasant, and normalizes response to stress. Treatment with more sustained steroids like prednisolone or dexamethasone is inadequate, as it exposes the patient to periods without any glucocorticoid at all. Fludrocortisone acetate treatment replaces aldosterone, providing a plasma renin activity comfortably within the range seen in health. Extra fludrocortisone is not required except in illness.

7.2. Lifestyle Modifications

Dietary adjustments can help manage Addison's disease. In general, a well-balanced diet containing fresh fruits, vegetables, whole grains, and protein sources is recommended. More information about special considerations for alternative diets and daily living can be found in Resources and FAQs. Smoking and the use of recreational drugs, including marijuana-based products, are generally discouraged due to the potential for detrimental effects. However, further studies are needed to understand the effects in individuals with Addison's disease. Reducing alcohol consumption promotes overall health and aids in preventing adrenal gland dysfunction. It is extremely important for individuals with adrenal insufficiency to avoid or at least limit excessive alcohol consumption. Weight management is an important part of a healthy lifestyle to reduce the influence of obesity-related illness on daily steroid requirements and to promote overall health. Nutritional changes can have an effect on overall health and potential cortisol needs. Supplement use should always be discussed with a healthcare provider to avoid interactions and negative effects. Individuals should generally consider inquiring with a healthcare provider about vitamin D supplements to maintain healthy levels, especially in regions without abundant natural sunlight. Moderately enjoying the sunshine is acceptable. Randomized control trials for optimal vitamin D levels in adrenal insufficiency have not been published. More detail about the role of vitamin D in adrenal insufficiency and supplements to consider can be found in the Vitamin D article by Grantham and Gay in the Resources section. It is generally recommended to limit caffeine for overall health benefits and effects on cortisol. It is also important to avoid excessive amounts, especially in the evening when trying to regulate sleep patterns. The overall safety of consuming green tea supplements or other herbal supplements in mild and moderate doses for individuals on hydrocortisone has not been reported scientifically in controlled scenarios at the time of publication. Some herbal products and a handful of available over-the-counter medications are known to interact with adrenal hormone replacement and should be used cautiously or avoided altogether. Patients should work with their doctor to discuss which over-the-counter medications or herbal supplements might be helpful or contraindicated in their situation. Always ensure healthcare providers are aware of all dietary supplements and over-the-counter and prescription medications taken by an individual on a regular basis. Massage, acupuncture, or other alternative therapies might be additional options to help with symptoms of fatigue and stress reduction. A person might consider discussing these alternatives with their healthcare providers. Balanced regular exercise is important to stay in good condition. In overcoming an illness or a severe stressor, the body will need medicinal doses of glucocorticoids. Regular physical activity will help keep the body healthy and strong. There are no formal guidelines around what exercise level or intensity an individual should do, and this should be a personal choice that ideally aligns with getting the approval of their doctor if they have specific conditions that might be adversely affected by exercise.

Addison's disease impacts the release of stress hormones. That's why lifestyle modifications, either by choice or requirement, are a significant aspect of treatment. As mistimed cortisol secretions can cause symptoms, maintaining a consistent daily routine is very important. It is recommended to avoid shift work and to get ample rest, especially during illness or significant stressors. It is also important for individuals to wear a medical alert necklace or bracelet and/or carry a medical alert card listing their diagnosis and emergency management plan in case of an emergency. Individuals may need to inform school and work personnel about their diagnosis and emergency management plans.

8. Complications and Prognosis

Alongside reactions to certain medications or anesthesia, it is also important to keep the following conditions in mind: Medication interactions. With Addison's disease, individuals must learn about steroids and how they affect other medications taken for unrelated health problems. It is necessary to discuss a complete list of medications with a medical professional, including over-the-counter and herbal medicines. Many over-the-counter and prescription medications can interfere with steroids. These can reduce cortisol levels to lower than what bodies need, leading to signs and symptoms described above. Parkinson's disease. Parkinson's disease and Addison's disease are usually caused by autoimmunity, so they are more common together. Usually only targeted testing for Addison's is necessary. Prognosis. With treatment, people with Addison's can live normal, healthy lives. They must learn to recognize signs of insufficient cortisol or aldosterone, like before sports competition. Given that Addison's is rare (with only 1 degree of separation), managing an Addison's disease health condition can be challenging due to the lack of widely accessible information and support.

Complications happen when an individual has untreated Addison's disease for a long time; sudden adrenal crisis can be life-threatening and require immediate medical attention. Addison's disease can also lead to other, usually minor, complications that can have a long-term impact on your health. Some of these include muscle weakness, which can cause difficulty walking, abdomen pains, low blood pressure when standing, extreme dizziness or fainting, and poor memory. The complications of Addison's disease can be caused by dehydration, low blood pressure, a low level of cortisol, or high levels of potassium in your blood. If left untreated, Addison's disease can lead to an adrenal crisis. This is a medical emergency in which people need immediate treatment to prevent problems such as heart failure. Surgery. Simple surgeries (like tooth extraction) can be more complicated due to the risks of general anesthesia and additional concerns resulting from the steroid replacement medication required. Pregnancy. Women with Addison's disease are at risk of having an adrenal crisis during pregnancy, so it's important to be closely managed by a healthcare provider while pregnant.

9. Research and Future Directions

The hope is that, eventually, researchers might find a combination of hormone-related gene activity that accurately indicates when an adrenal gland is in distress. Professor Greg Anderson at the Centre for Endocrinology, Diabetes and Metabolism in Birmingham is also hopeful that genomic sequencing research could in the future transform care for people with Addison's. "Advances in genomics may allow unique 'omic' profiles which could predict individuals' biological responses to particular hormone replacement agents," he says. Professor John Wass, from the John Radcliffe Hospital in Oxford, studies the long-term effects of Addison's. While we hope to learn the results of this study soon, he also says, "Addison's sufferers, when diagnosed, appropriately worry about salt, excessive or insufficient. We shall clarify this routinely prevalent issue by studying the quality of bone, the risk of kidney stones in Addison's disease. We will complement this with studies of life and if people with Addison's who take specific medications have a better quality of life."

There are no ongoing clinical trials in the UK at present. In the future, researchers believe that an "artificial" or lab-made version of the ACTH hormone might be used to diagnose Addison's. According to the team at University College London/Royal Free Hospital, "It's increasingly clear that, while autoantibody tests are important, there is also a failure to make the correct diagnosis in patients as the symptoms of other conditions can mimic those of adrenal insufficiency. We term these 'mis-diagnosis by over-diagnosis' as they lead many healthy patients to have at best unnecessary and at worst harmful treatments."